Dr. Utipmfon Sukmama Jimmy

OCCUPATIONAL MEDICINE

ISBN
Hardbound-978-621-495-038-6
MOBI/KINDLE-978-621-495-039-3
Softbound/Paperback-978-621-495-040-9

Published by:
Poetry Planet Book Publishing House
Rosario Pozorrubio, Pangasinan, Philippines
Contact Number: +639554960094
Email: maritesritumalta@gmail.com

TABLE OF CONTENTS

PREFACE

In today's world, when the health and safety of workers are of the utmost importance to companies, governments, and society as a whole, occupational medicine is a field that bears a tremendous amount of relevance. Because of the constant evolution of workplaces and the emergence of new issues, there has never been a time when there was a greater need for a complete understanding and management of occupational health risks.

This book, titled "Occupational Medicine: A Comprehensive Guide to Workplace Health and Safety," is intended to serve as a definitive reference for individuals working in the field of occupational medicine as well as students who are already enrolled in the subject. It discusses a wide variety of subjects, ranging from the origins and development of occupational health to the evaluation and management of occupational diseases and hazards.

Starting with the fundamentals, such as the definition and scope of the subject, and then delving into more specialized areas, such as occupational dangers, diseases, and health promotion, the chapters in this book are organized in such a way as to provide a comprehensive overview of occupational medicine. The information that is presented in each chapter has been painstakingly researched and prepared by professionals in the industry. This ensures that the information is correct, up to date, and pertinent to the practice that is currently being used.

The fact that this book places such an emphasis on practical applications is one of its most notable characteristics. The reader will find real-world examples, case studies, and practical ideas that may be utilized in the workplace throughout the chapters of the book. There is something that this book can provide for you, regardless of whether you are an experienced occupational health expert or a student who is just beginning their career in the industry.

For the purpose of making this book a reality, I would like to express my appreciation to the contributors who have kindly offered their knowledge and skills. My hope is that it will be a useful resource for anybody who is interested in occupational medicine and that it will help to the improvement of workplace health and safety all over the world because of its contributions.

I

INTRODUCTION

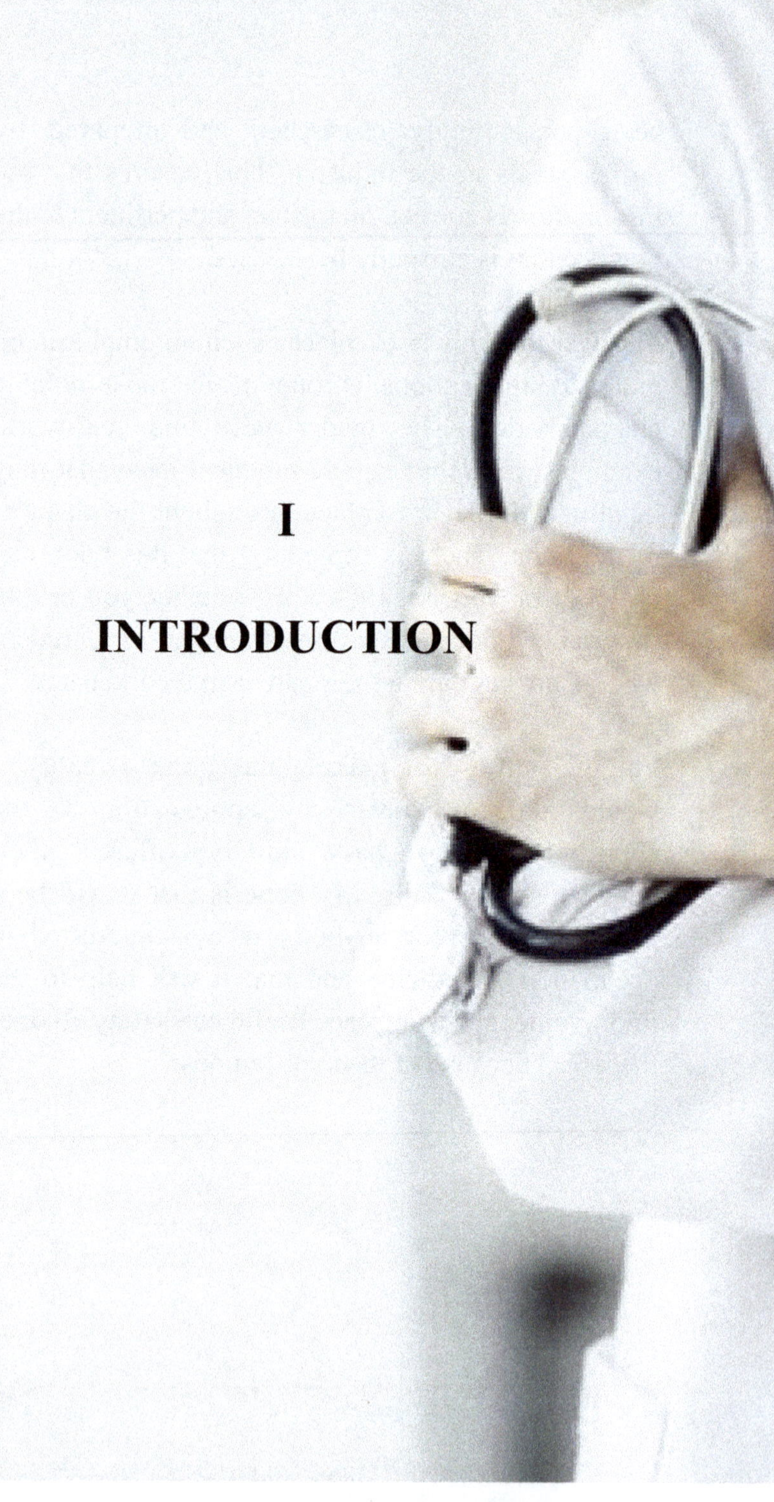

Definition and Scope of Occupational Medicine

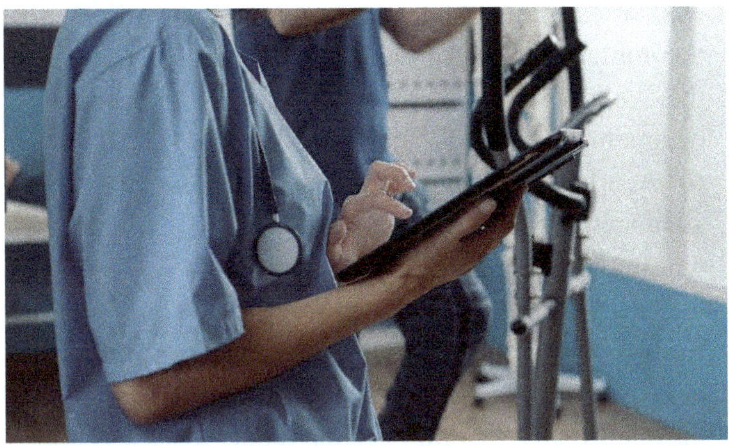

Occupational medicine is a distinct field of medicine that specifically addresses the physical and mental health of individuals working in a certain environment. The field includes various areas of study, such as preventative medicine, clinical care, rehabilitation, and occupational health and safety. Occupational medicine experts, also known as occupational health physicians, have a vital responsibility in promoting the safe and efficient performance of workers' tasks, while simultaneously mitigating the potential for work-related injuries and illnesses.

The field of occupational medicine encompasses a wide range of specialties that pertain to the domains of workplace health and safety. The aforementioned activities encompass the identification and evaluation of potential dangers within the workplace, the implementation of medical monitoring to oversee the well-being of employees who are exposed to occupational hazards, the provision of medical care for work-related injuries and illnesses, and the advancement of health and wellness initiatives within the workplace.

Early detection and intervention are crucial objectives in the field of occupational medicine, as they aim to prevent occupational diseases and injuries. This objective is accomplished through a range of strategies, encompassing risk evaluation, health instruction, and the formulation of policies and initiatives aimed at fostering a secure and conducive work milieu.

Occupational medicine is of paramount importance in the rehabilitation process for individuals who have sustained injuries or developed illnesses as a result of their occupational activities. This may encompass the provision of medical intervention, rehabilitation interventions, and support in facilitating a safe and prompt reintegration into the workforce.

Workplace medicine specialists engage in collaborative efforts with employers, workers, and government agencies to formulate and execute policies and initiatives aimed at enhancing workplace health and safety, in addition to delivering direct medical care. The aforementioned activities encompass the performance of workplace inspections, the provision of training and education pertaining to occupational health and safety matters, and the active promotion of enhanced working conditions.

In its whole, occupational medicine is an indispensable and ever-evolving domain that assumes a pivotal function in safeguarding and advancing the physical and mental welfare of employees. Occupational health and safety (OHS) comprises a diverse array of fields and endeavors that are focused on maintaining the safe and efficient performance of workers, while simultaneously mitigating the potential for work-related accidents and diseases. In the subsequent parts, a comprehensive examination of occupational medicine will be undertaken, encompassing its historical background, fundamental principles, and contemporary methodologies.

Importance of Occupational Health and Safety

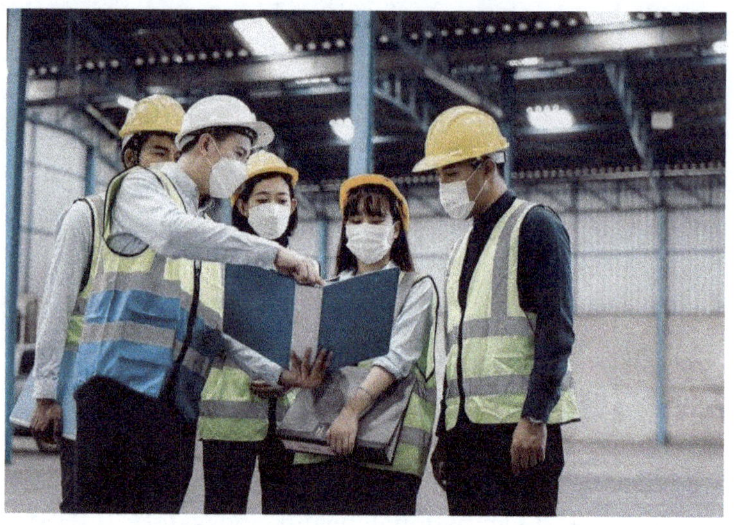

Occupational health and safety (OHS) is a vital component of workplace administration that seeks to safeguard the well-being, security, and physical condition of employees. Occupational health and safety initiatives involve a diverse array of actions and practices that are designed to mitigate workplace accidents and injuries, while also diminishing the likelihood of work-related illnesses and disorders. The significance of Occupational Health and Safety (OHS) cannot be exaggerated, as it not only safeguards employees but also carries wider ramifications for organizations, society, and the overall economy.

The significance of Occupational Health and Safety (OHS) lies in its role in mitigating occupational injuries and diseases. OHS programmes have the capacity to diminish the likelihood of accidents and injuries, thereby fostering a safer work environment for all employees, through the identification and mitigation of workplace risks. Implementing this measure not only safeguards employees against potential injury but also mitigates the economic and societal burdens linked to workplace accidents and injuries.

In addition to mitigating the occurrence of injuries and diseases, occupational health and safety (OHS) also assumes a pivotal role in fostering the overall health and welfare of workers. OHS programmes have the potential to enhance the overall health and quality of life of workers by addressing several variables that may lead to poor health, including exposure to hazardous substances, ergonomic dangers, and psychosocial stresses. Consequently, this can result in heightened efficiency, decreased rates of employee absences, and enhanced staff morale.

Moreover, Occupational Health and Safety (OHS) plays a crucial role in guaranteeing adherence to legal and regulatory obligations. Numerous nations have implemented legal frameworks and regulatory measures mandating employers to ensure the provision of a secure and conducive work environment for their workforce. Noncompliance with these stipulations may lead to financial penalties, legal proceedings, and harm to the organization's standing. Through the implementation of efficient occupational health and safety (OHS) programmes, organizations may guarantee adherence to these regulations and prevent possible legal and financial repercussions.

Occupational Health and Safety (OHS) also assumes a crucial role in safeguarding the environment and the community. Inadequate management of industrial dangers, such as perilous chemicals and pollutants, can detrimentally affect the environment and the neighboring community. Organizations can mitigate their environmental effect and promote a safer and healthier community by developing occupational health and safety (OHS) programmes that specifically target these hazards.

Ensuring Occupational Health and Safety (OHS) is of paramount significance. Workplace management is a crucial element that serves the dual purpose of safeguarding employees and yielding wider ramifications for organizations, society, and the economy. OHS programmes are essential for establishing secure, healthy, and sustainable workplaces by preventing accidents and diseases, promoting health and well-being, ensuring adherence to legal obligations, and safeguarding the environment.

II.

HISTORY OF OCCUPATIONAL MEDICINE

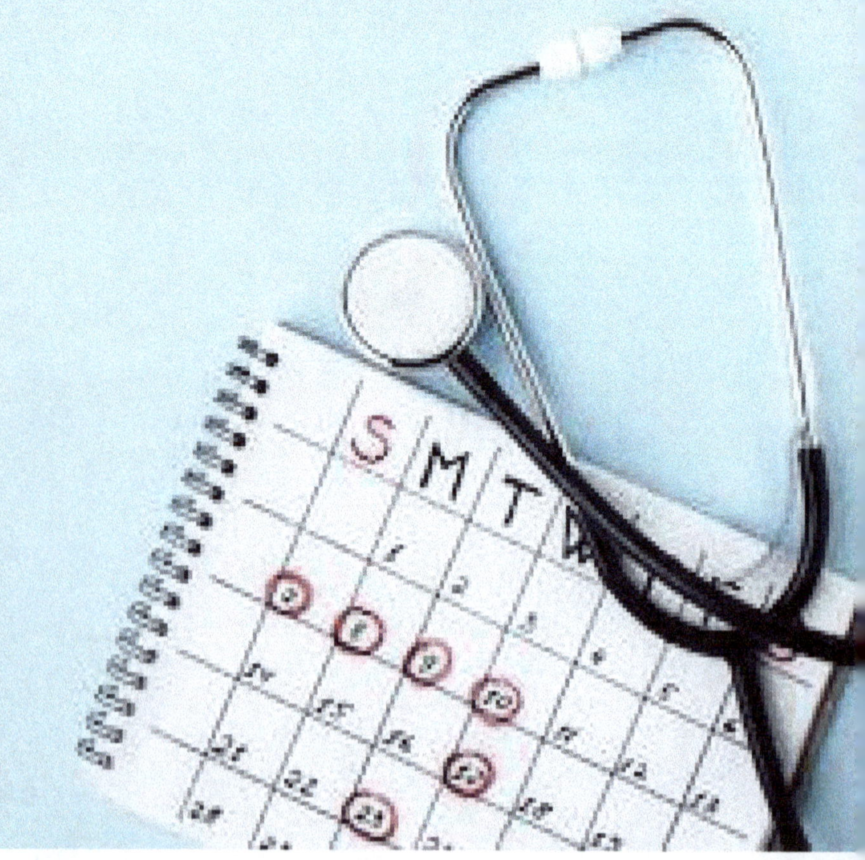

A. Origins and Evolution

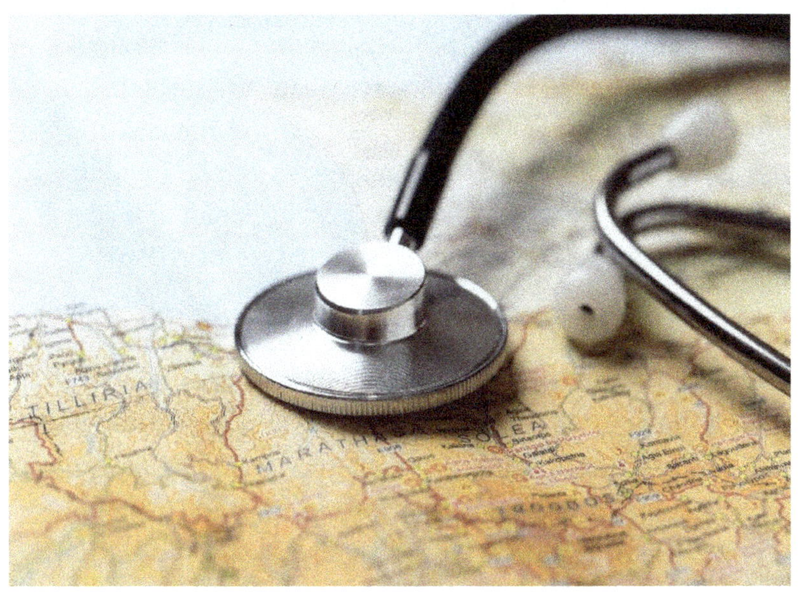

Occupational medicine, a multidisciplinary discipline that has developed from ancient civilizations' fundamental practices to the present-day concerns of worker health and safety in industries, boasts an extensive historical lineage spanning centuries. The concept of this can be historically linked to early human societies, during which members of society acknowledged the correlation between occupational tasks and health results.

Ancient civilizations, including Egypt, Greece, and Rome, implemented occupational health practices in their most basic forms. Personnel in these societies were exposed to a wide array of occupational hazards, including physical harm and noxious substance exposure. Indicative of an early awareness of occupational health issues, references to occupational injuries and treatments can be found in ancient texts, including the Edwin Smith Papyrus originating from ancient Egypt.

Guilds arose as significant institutions during the Middle Ages to regulate and safeguard the interests of laborers. Guilds provided their members with fundamental forms of support and healthcare, including treatment for workplace injuries. However, these early endeavors frequently lacked scientific rigor and had a restricted scope.

During the 18th and 19th centuries, the industrial revolution occurred, which signified a pivotal moment in the development of occupational medicine. The exponential expansion of manufacturing facilities and industrial output precipitated a notable upsurge in occupational ailments and injuries. During this era, perilous working conditions emerged, including prolonged work hours, contact with hazardous equipment, and inhalation of toxic substances like lead and coal dust.

Governments and employers began to acknowledge the necessity of institutionalized approaches to occupational health and safety as a reaction to these challenges. The earliest documented occurrence of legislation designed to safeguard the welfare of workers occurred in Britain during the 1700s, when the Factory Acts were enacted. By enacting these laws, child labor was restricted and fundamental safety standards were instituted in factories.

Occupational medicine experienced notable progressions throughout the 20th century, propelled by scientific revelations, technological developments, and social movements that championed the rights of workers. A critical juncture in the annals of occupational medicine was the Triangle Shirtwaist Factory fire of 1911, an incident that tragically claimed the lives of 146 garment workers situated in New York City. As a result of the public outrage that this calamity evoked, new labor laws and regulations were enacted with the intention of enhancing health and safety in the workplace.

Organizations such as the International Commission on Occupational Health (ICOH) in 1950 and the American College of Occupational and Environmental Medicine (ACOEM) in 1916 further advanced the development of occupational medicine over the course of the 20th century. These organizations significantly contributed to the progression of occupational medicine by means of their efforts in advocacy, education, and research.

During the latter half of the 20th century, occupational medicine's contribution to addressing emergent health challenges in the workplace became increasingly apparent. Chemical exposure, ergonomic injuries, and psychosocial stress emerged as matters of growing significance in the attention of occupational health practitioners. A greater variety of disciplines were incorporated into the field as it grew in scope, such as industrial hygiene, toxicology, epidemiology, and behavioral science.

Occupational medicine encountered novel challenges and prospects during the late 20th and early 21st centuries due to the expansion of globalization and technological progress. The outsourcing of manufacturing processes and the globalization of supply chains have generated apprehensions regarding labor rights and working conditions in developing nations. Concurrently, advancements in telemedicine and information technology created novel opportunities for the remote provision of occupational health services.

Presently, occupational medicine is an expansive and ever-evolving discipline that covers a vast array of endeavors with the objective of safeguarding and advancing the health and welfare of personnel. Occupational health professionals are employed in corporations, clinics, hospitals, and government agencies, among other contexts. They are responsible for implementing medical treatment and rehabilitation services for injured workers, conducting risk assessments, and devising workplace interventions; thus, they play a crucial role in preventing workplace illnesses and injuries.

Modern occupational medicine encompasses not only conventional occupational hazards, including chemical exposures and physical injuries, but also emerging concerns including exhaustion, work-related stress, and the health consequences of sedentary lifestyles. Occupational health professionals devise and implement strategies for establishing safe and healthy workplaces in collaboration with employers, labor unions, government agencies, and other stakeholders.

Occupational medicine will likely continue to develop in the future in response to technological advancements, changes in the nature of work, and societal attitudes toward health and safety. The advent of automation, the freelance economy, and remote work will give rise to novel prospects and challenges, necessitating the implementation of inventive methodologies and interdisciplinary alliances to safeguard the physical and mental welfare of employees throughout the twenty-first century and beyond.

Milestones in Occupational Health Legislation

Occupational health legislation has been instrumental in safeguarding the rights of workers, fostering a secure work environment, and mitigating the occurrence of occupational illnesses and injuries. At different points in time, legislative developments have constituted pivotal moments in history, exerting a profound influence on workplace procedures and the relative importance that employers and workers place on health and safety. The following are significant turning points in occupational health legislation:

1. Factory Acts (18th-19th centuries): In response to the hazardous working conditions in factories during the Industrial Revolution, the United Kingdom enacted a series of laws known as the Factory Acts between the 18th and 19th centuries. The purpose of these acts was to prevent child labor, restrict working hours, and mandate ventilation and guardrail installation on machinery, among other fundamental safety measures for industrial facilities.

2. United States: Occupational Safety and Health Act (OSHA) of 1970 OSHA is a seminal legislation that established the Occupational Safety and Health Administration (OSHA) under the Department of Labor in the United States. The primary objective of OSHA is to guarantee healthful and secure working environments for employees through the establishment and enforcement of regulations, provision of training, outreach, education, and support. The Act applies to certain public sector employers and employees in the 50 states, certain territories, and jurisdictions under federal authority, in addition to the majority of private sector employers and employees.

3. The 1974 Health and Safety in the Workplace Act (United Kingdom): The principal legislative instrument that regulates occupational health and safety in the United Kingdom is the Health and Safety at Work Act 1974. Employers are obligated by law to ensure the well-being, health, and safety of their workforce, in addition to any third parties who may be impacted by their operations. The Health and Safety Executive (HSE) was designated by the Act as the regulatory authority tasked with the enforcement of health and safety standards in the workplace.

4. The 1994 Malaysian Occupational Safety and Health Act: In Malaysia, the Occupational Safety and Health Act 1994 is an all-encompassing statute designed to uphold and encourage the utmost level of occupational safety and health standards across all work environments. Employers are obligated to ensure a secure working environment, conduct risk assessments, and implement preventative measures against occupational diseases and accidents. The Act additionally designates the Department of Occupational Safety and Health (DOSH) as the regulatory body tasked with the enforcement of standards pertaining to occupational health and safety.

5. European Framework Directive on Safety and Health at Work (1989): Adopted in 1989, the European Framework Directive on Safety and Health at Work establishes overarching principles pertaining to the safeguarding of workers' health and safety within the European Union and the prevention of occupational hazards. It mandates that EU member states implement risk assessments, preventative measures, and training programs to ensure that employers take appropriate precautions to safeguard the health and safety of their employees.

The aforementioned legislative landmarks in occupational health demonstrate an increasing acknowledgment of the significance of safety in the workplace and the necessity for all-encompassing legal structures that safeguard the health and welfare of employees. Although considerable advancements have been achieved thus far, continuous endeavors are required to tackle emerging occupational health issues and guarantee that every worker is provided with secure and healthy work environments.

III.

OCCUPATIONAL HAZARD

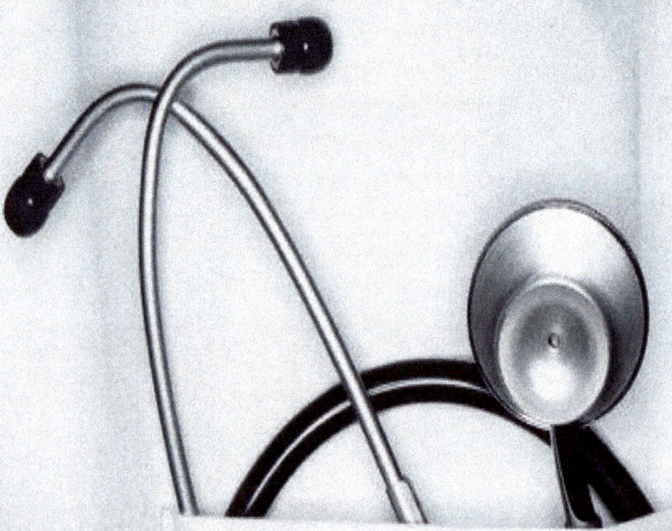

Occupational hazards in medicine comprise a multitude of potential dangers that healthcare practitioners encounter in the course of their routine professional duties. There are four primary categories into which these hazards can be classified: physical, chemical, biological, and psychosocial. Every category poses distinct obstacles and necessitates particular approaches to alleviate hazards and guarantee the well-being and security of healthcare personnel.

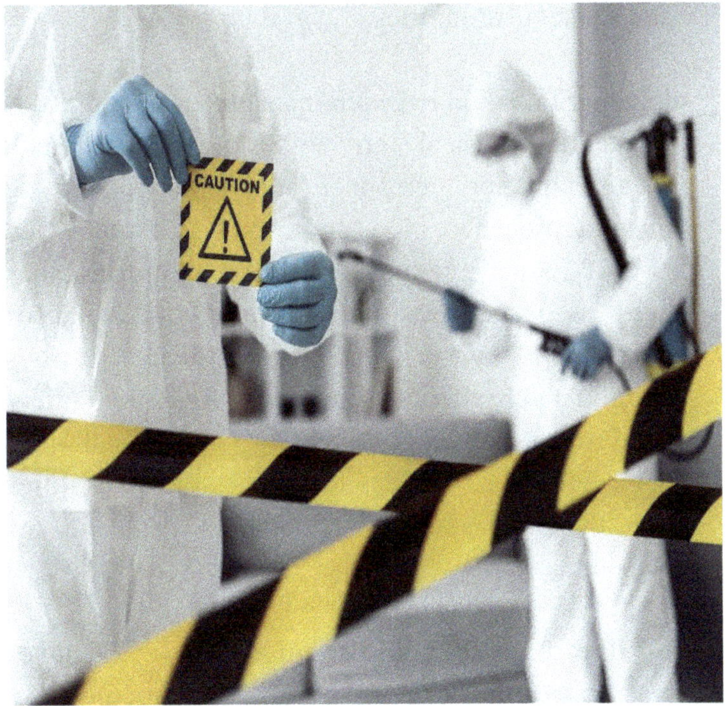

A. Physical Hazards

Physical hazards in medicine pertain to perils that emerge from the tangible surroundings or apparatus utilized within healthcare environments. Injuries including musculoskeletal disorders, slides, trips, falls, and ergonomic injuries may result from these dangers. Healthcare practitioners frequently perform physically strenuous duties, including patient transfers and lifting, which, if not executed with appropriate technique, may result in muscle strain and subsequent injuries.

Ionizing radiation exposure constitutes an additional substantial physical peril within the medical field, specifically for personnel conducting diagnostic imaging procedures like fluoroscopy, CT scans, and X-rays. Extended exposure to ionizing radiation has been associated with an elevated likelihood of developing cancer and experiencing various detrimental health consequences. Radiation safety measures, including shielding and monitoring devices, must be implemented in healthcare facilities to reduce the danger of radiation exposure for personnel.

Healthcare professionals may also encounter instances of violence and aggression perpetrated by patients or their relatives, with a particular emphasis on emergency departments and psychiatric facilities. Injuries inflicted during physical assaults may vary in severity, spanning from minor lacerations and bruising to more profound trauma. To protect healthcare workers from workplace violence, hospitals and healthcare organizations should implement security measures, such as training personnel in de-escalation techniques and providing crisis buttons or emergency response systems.

B. Chemical Hazards

Exposure to hazardous substances, including disinfectants, sterilizing agents, chemotherapy drugs, and hazardous drugs utilized in pharmaceutical compounding, constitutes chemical hazards in medicine. Long-term health effects, including cancer and reproductive disorders, and skin irritation, respiratory issues, and allergic reactions, may be experienced by healthcare personnel who come into contact with these substances.

It is critical to avoid exposure to hazardous substances in healthcare settings through the implementation of appropriate procedures for their storage, disposal, and handling. To reduce the risk of chemical exposure among healthcare personnel, facilities should provide appropriate personal protective equipment (PPE), including goggles, respirators, and gloves, and implement safe handling procedures and ventilation systems.

C. Biological Hazards

Biological hazards in medicine result from infectious agent exposure, including that caused by bacteria, viruses, fungi, and parasites. Biological hazards can potentially be encountered by healthcare personnel via their handling of patients' blood, bodily fluids, tissues, and contaminated medical devices. Healthcare-associated infections (HAIs) can result from occupational exposure to biological hazards, posing a substantial risk to both healthcare personnel and patients.

Standard precautions must be observed to prevent occupational exposure to biological hazards; these include practicing safe injection techniques, maintaining hand hygiene, and donning personal protective equipment (PPE) such as gowns, masks, gloves, and eye protection. In addition to providing vaccinations and post-exposure prophylaxis, healthcare facilities should implement infection control measures, including environmental cleansing and disinfection, to safeguard healthcare personnel against occupational exposures and vaccine-preventable diseases.

D. Psychosocial Hazards

Psychosocial hazards in medicine pertain to elements of the physical, mental, and social domains of the healthcare profession that have the potential to impact the health and well-being of personnel. High workload, extended working hours, shift work, job-related stress, workplace violence, bullying, harassment, and burnout are examples of these dangers. A variety of adverse effects, including anxiety, depression, fatigue, insomnia, substance misuse, and suicidal ideation, may be exacerbated by psychosocial hazards.

To effectively mitigate psychosocial hazards, a comprehensive strategy is necessary, taking into account organizational and individual factors. It is imperative for healthcare organizations to foster a nurturing work environment, furnish stress management and mental health support resources, and execute approaches that enhance work-life equilibrium while mitigating job demands and burden. In addition, programming that focuses on violence prevention, conflict resolution, and communication skills can assist healthcare professionals in managing psychosocial hazards in the workplace.

Medical occupational hazards present substantial threats to the health and safety of healthcare personnel. Healthcare institutions can safeguard the health and safety of their personnel and establish more secure work environments by identifying and addressing the various types of risks associated with them. In healthcare settings, occupational health and safety must take precedence over all else in order to guarantee that personnel can maintain delivering superior care while reducing their exposure to occupational illnesses and injuries.

IV.

OCCUPATIONAL DISEASES

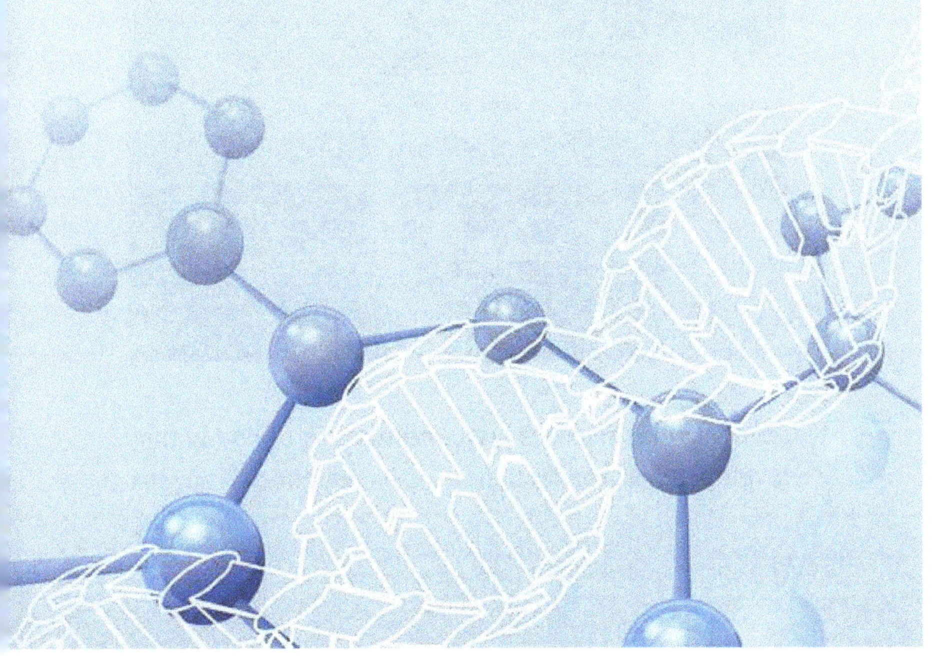

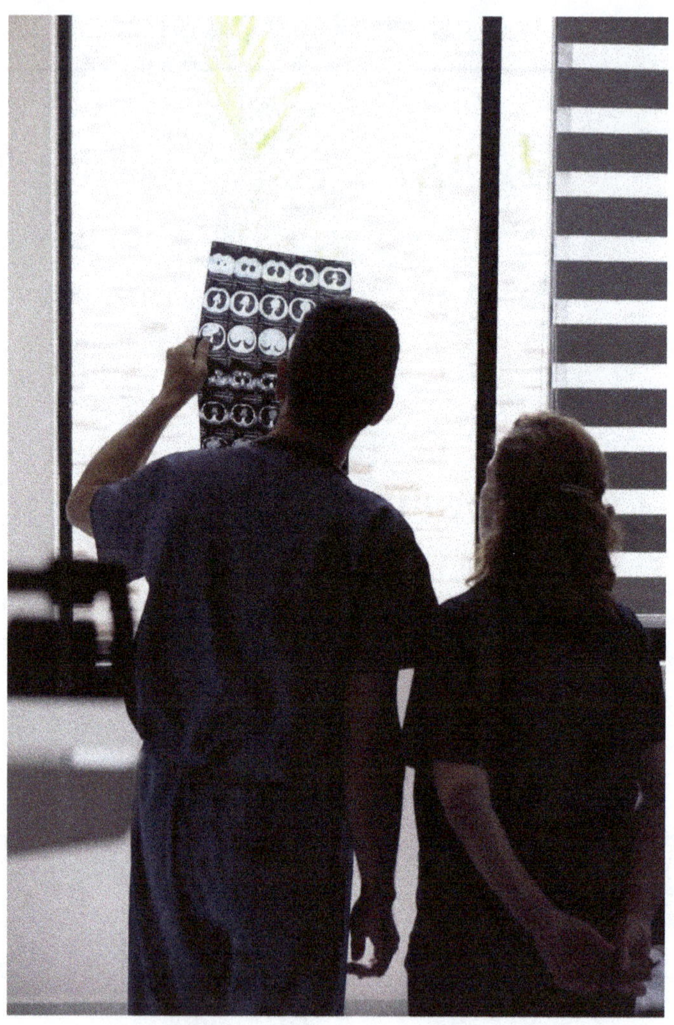

Occupational diseases are conditions of the body that develop as a consequence of occupational hazard exposure. Although the precise hazards differ contingent upon the demands of the task at hand, certain ailments are frequently linked to particular vocations and sectors. It is critical to comprehend these prevalent occupational diseases in order to safeguard the health of employees and prevent maladies that may occur in the workplace.

1. Respiratory Diseases: Biological agents, dust, and occupational pollutants have the potential to cause respiratory ailments in personnel, including pneumoconiosis, chronic obstructive pulmonary disease (COPD), and occupational asthma. Sectors including manufacturing, construction, mining, and construction are especially vulnerable to the detrimental effects of chemical vapors, dust, and emissions.

2. Skin Disorders: Skin disorders, including contact dermatitis, eczema, and irritants, allergens, and hazardous substances, may result from exposed skin. Mechanics, food transporters, healthcare professionals, and hairdressers are all susceptible to developing skin disorders as a result of their contact with detergents, latex, and chemicals.

3. Hearing Loss: Extended occupational noise exposure may result in the development of hearing impairment, tinnitus, and additional auditory conditions. A number of sectors, including manufacturing, construction, mining, and agriculture, frequently produce noise-damaging environments in which employees operate without appropriate hearing protection.

4. Musculoskeletal Disorders (MSDs): Musculoskeletal disorders, including but not limited to carpal tunnel syndrome, tendonitis, and lower back discomfort, may be induced by awkward postures, routine motions, excessive weight bearing, and ergonomic risks. MSDs are prevalent among employees in construction, manufacturing, nursing, and assembly line labor.

5. Occupational Cancer: Ionizing radiation, asbestos, benzene, formaldehyde, and other carcinogens can increase the risk of developing occupational malignancies including bladder cancer, mesothelioma, lung cancer, and leukemia. During the course of their work, employees in industries including mining, construction, healthcare,

and manufacturing may be exposed to carcinogenic substances.

B. Emerging Occupational Health Concerns

Apart from the aforementioned prevalent occupational diseases, there are nascent occupational health issues that are garnering considerable interest as a result of evolving workplace hazards, technological progress, and shifting work practices.

1. Psychosocial Health: The recognition of mental health concerns, including but not limited to stress, anxiety, melancholy, and burnout, as substantial occupational health issues, is growing. Poor work-life balance, work-related stress, and high job demands can all contribute to negative mental health outcomes among employees in a variety of industries.

2. Emerging Infectious Diseases: In healthcare settings and other high-risk occupations, the emergence of novel infectious diseases such as COVID-19 emphasizes the significance of infection control measures and occupational health preparedness. Healthcare professionals, first responders, and essential personnel may encounter heightened hazards

of encountering infectious agents in the course of pandemics and outbreaks.

3. Work-related Musculoskeletal Disorders (WRMSDs): As the prevalence of technology adoption and sedentary work environments increase, so does concern regarding the occurrence of work-related musculoskeletal disorders (WRMSDs), including repetitive strain injuries, neck pain, and back pain. Sedentary occupations and prolonged seating, inadequate ergonomics, and repetitive computer use are factors that contribute to WRMSDs among office workers.

4. Emerging Chemical Exposures: New substances and chemicals have been introduced into the workplace as a result of technological advancements and modifications to manufacturing processes, raising concerns about potential health dangers to employees. Nanomaterials, pharmaceuticals, electronic detritus, and flame retardants are a few examples of emerging chemical exposures.

5. Climate-related Health Hazards: Extreme weather events and climate change present new occupational health risks, especially for

those who work outdoors or in sectors including emergency response, construction, agriculture, and construction. Natural disasters, heat stress, air pollution, and vector-borne diseases are a few of the climate-related health risks that may threaten the health and safety of laborers.

A comprehensive understanding of prevalent occupational illnesses as well as emergent occupational health issues is critical in fostering a secure and health-conscious workplace. In order to safeguard the health and safety of employees across all sectors, employers, policymakers, and healthcare practitioners can collectively resolve occupational health challenges through the identification of potential hazards, implementation of preventative measures, and promotion of education and awareness.

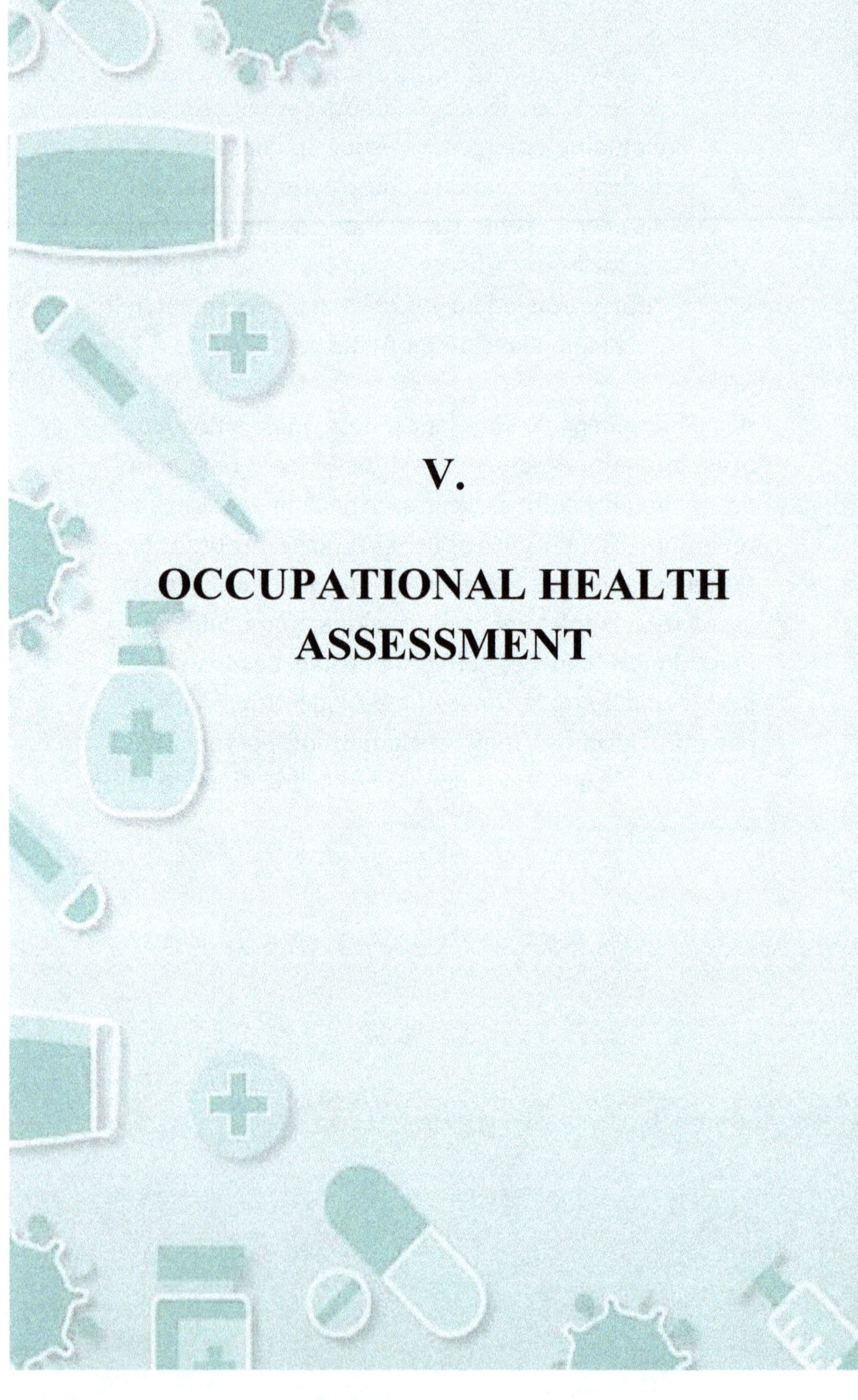

V.

OCCUPATIONAL HEALTH ASSESSMENT

The occupational health assessment procedure is an essential undertaking that seeks to appraise and oversee the physical and mental welfare of employees across diverse sectors. The process entails the collection of data regarding the medical backgrounds of employees, the execution of physical assessments, and the administration of screening examinations in order to detect possible occupational health hazards and avert work-related ailments and injuries. Employers can foster a secure and healthful work environment and benefit the general welfare of their personnel by implementing an all-encompassing strategy for occupational health assessment.

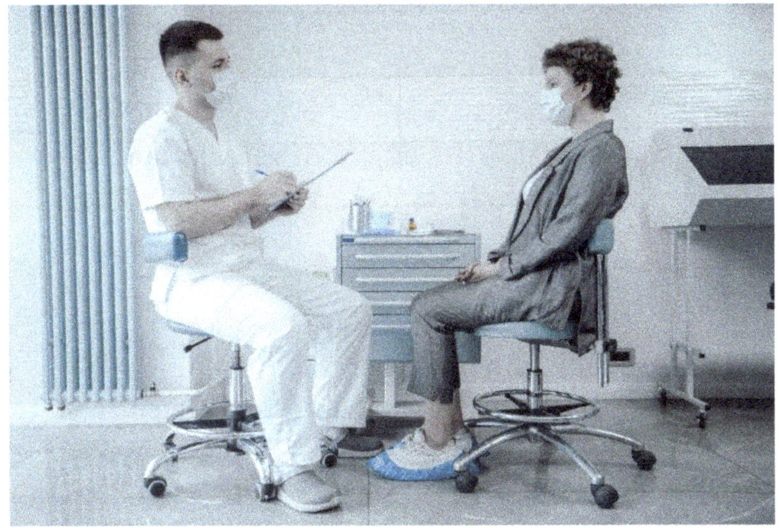

A. Occupational Health History

The occupational health history is an essential element of the evaluation procedure, as it furnishes significant data regarding the previous and present health condition of the employee, occupational health issues, and work-related hazards. Healthcare practitioners gather data regarding the subsequent topics during the occupational health history interview:

1. Work History: Collecting information regarding the positions, responsibilities, and work environments of employees aids in the detection of potential occupational risks and the evaluation of the likelihood of work-related maladies and injuries. To comprehend the nature of workers' exposures and their potential health effects, it is critical to have knowledge regarding their previous and current occupations, industries, and job duties.

2. Health History: Gaining insight into the medical backgrounds of employees, encompassing previous injuries, maladies, and chronic ailments, enables healthcare practitioners to detect pre-existing conditions that could potentially compromise the safety

of job performance. Additionally, knowledge of a family medical history, medications, surgeries, and allergies can offer valuable insights into the general health condition of employees and identify potential risk factors that may contribute to work-related health issues.

3. Exposure History: Exploring the extent to which employees are exposed to ergonomic hazards, noise, vibration, and occupational hazards, aids in the identification of potential origins of occupational health risks. Inquiries pertaining to work-related accidents, injuries, and near misses may additionally yield valuable information regarding the extent of workers' exposure and the efficacy of current safety protocols.

4. Symptoms and Complaints: Exploring the extent to which employees are exposed to ergonomic hazards, noise, vibration, and occupational hazards, aids in the identification of potential origins of occupational health risks. Inquiries pertaining to work-related accidents, injuries, and near misses may additionally yield valuable information regarding the extent of

workers' exposure and the efficacy of current safety protocols.

5. Health Behaviors and Lifestyle Factors: By investigating the coping mechanisms, lifestyle factors, and health behaviors of employees, healthcare professionals can gain insight into how these elements may impact the health outcomes of employees and their capacity to effectively manage occupational health risks. Strategies for reducing occupational health hazards and promoting healthier behaviors may be informed by data regarding smoking, alcohol consumption, diet, exercise routines, and stress management techniques.

B. Physical Examination in the Workplace

The implementation of physical examinations within the workplace setting enables healthcare practitioners to evaluate the general health condition of employees, identify preliminary indications of occupational health complications, and detect work-related ailments and injuries. The physical examination may comprise the subsequent elements:

1. General Examination: An evaluation of the general appearance, vital signs (including blood pressure, pulse rate, and temperature), and overall physical condition of employees yields valuable information regarding their health status as a whole and possible indications of illness or injury.

2. Respiratory Examination: Lung auscultation, percussion, and spirometry testing are utilized to evaluate the respiratory function of employees. This aids in the detection of respiratory ailments such as chronic obstructive pulmonary disease (COPD), pneumoconiosis, and occupational asthma.

3. Musculoskeletal Examination: Musculoskeletal disorders, including back pain, repetitive strain injuries, and ergonomic-related issues, can be detected through the evaluation of workers' posture, range of motion, strength, and coordination.

4. Dermatological Examination: The assessment of workers' skin for indications of inflammation, irritation, rash, or dermatitis serves to detect possible skin disorders that may be associated with occupational

exposures to allergens, chemicals, or other perilous substances.

5. Neurological Examination: The evaluation of employees' neurological capabilities, encompassing assessments of their motor skills, sensory perception, and reflexes, serves to detect indications of neurological disorders such as vibration-induced white finger, carpal tunnel syndrome, and peripheral neuropathy.

C. Occupational Health Screening

The purpose of occupational health screening tests is to evaluate the health status of employees, identify early indicators of occupational illnesses and injuries, and track the efficacy of preventative measures implemented in the work environment. The following are typical occupational health monitoring tests:

1. Spirometry: Lung function is evaluated and respiratory conditions such as occupational asthma, COPD, and pneumoconiosis are identified via spirometry.

2. Audiometry: Hearing function is evaluated and hearing loss, tinnitus, and other auditory disorders associated with occupational noise exposure are identified through audiometry testing.

3. Vision Evaluation: Vision evaluation identifies visual impairments and eye disorders associated with occupational hazards, such as chemical exposure, eye fatigue, and glare, through the assessment of visual acuity, color vision, and visual field.

4. Blood Tests: Specific biomarkers, complete blood count (CBC), liver function tests (LFTs), and kidney function tests are among the blood tests that aid in determining the overall health status of employees and identify occupational diseases in their nascent stages, including lead toxicity, liver damage, and kidney dysfunction.

5. Biological Monitoring: Biological monitoring encompasses the assessment of employees' exposure levels to perilous substances via blood, urine, or other biological samples, including but not limited to heavy metals, pesticides, solvents, and biological agents. Biological monitoring is a

valuable tool utilized to evaluate the efficacy of control measures, ascertain the early stages of occupational diseases, and ascertain the actual exposure levels of workers.

Occupational health assessment is of the utmost importance in safeguarding the welfare of employees, preventing work-related ailments and injuries, and promoting health and safety in the workplace. Through the utilization of exhaustive occupational health histories, physical examinations, and screening tests, healthcare practitioners are capable of discerning potential hazards to employee health, implementing suitable preventive measures, and promoting the general welfare and health of personnel across all sectors.

VI.

OCCUPATIONAL HEALTH AND SAFETY MANAGEMENT

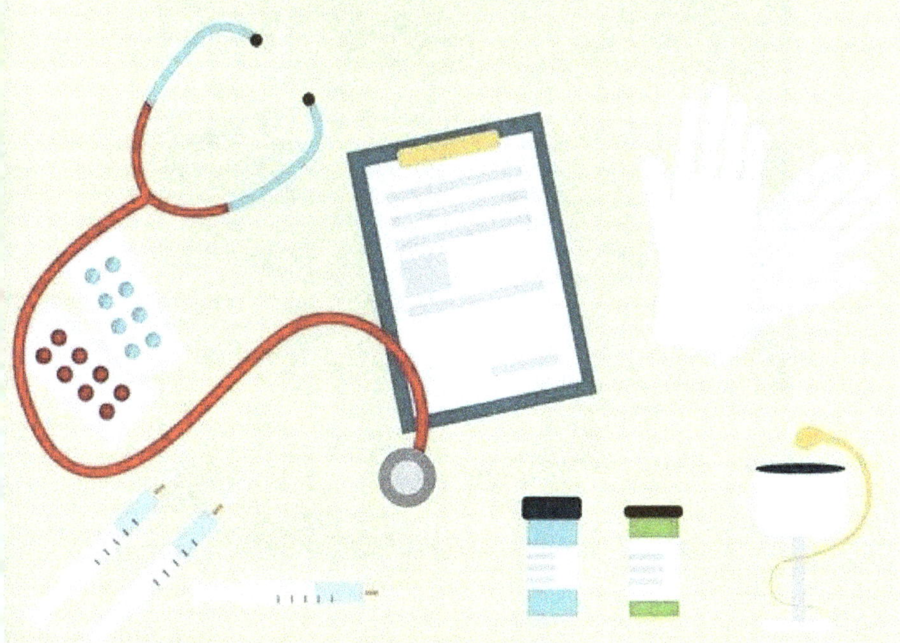

Management of occupational health and safety (OHS) is critical for safeguarding the health and safety of employees and ensuring a secure workplace. Organizations can minimize hazards, prevent work-related injuries and illnesses, and enhance the general health and well-being of their employees by implementing efficient risk assessment and management strategies, developing comprehensive occupational health programs and policies, and advocating for ergonomics in the workplace.

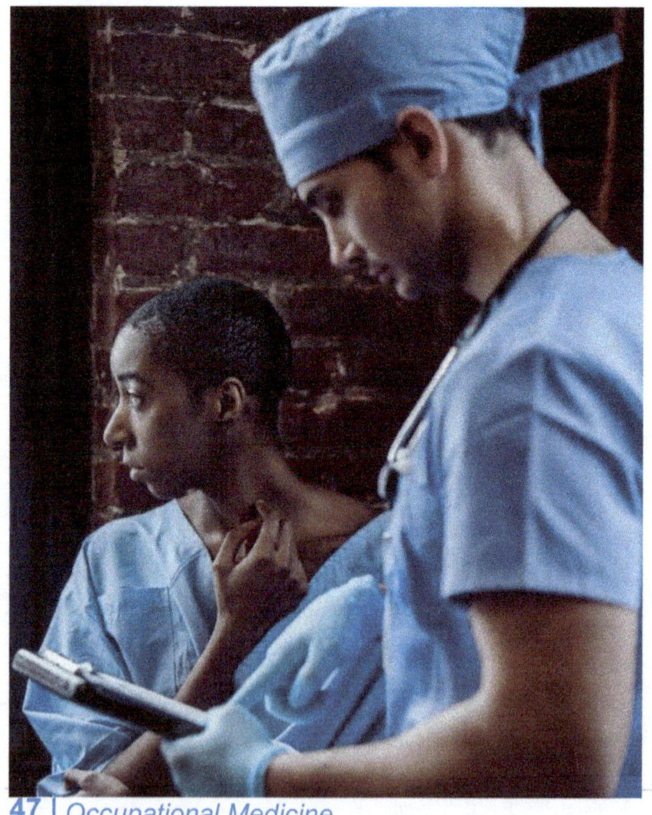

A. Evaluation and Management of Risks

OHS management is predicated on risk assessment and management, which entails the identification, evaluation, and control of hazards in the workplace in order to mitigate the potential for worker injury. A risk assessment and management procedure comprises the subsequent stages:

1. Identifying potential workplace hazards constitutes the initial phase of the risk assessment methodology. Physical, chemical, biological, ergonomic, and psychosocial elements that pose a threat to the health and safety of employees are examples of hazards.

2. Risk Assessment: The process of evaluating the probability and severity of damage linked to every identified hazard is crucial for the prioritization of risks and the identification of suitable control measures. Risk assessment entails taking into account various elements, including the characteristics of the peril, the extent of exposure, the vulnerability of personnel, and the possible ramifications of said exposure.

3. Control Measures It is essential to implement control measures to eliminate or reduce hazards in the workplace in order to prevent occupational illnesses and injuries. Personal protective equipment (e.g., respirators, eyewear, and engineering controls), administrative controls (e.g., training, work procedures, and signage), and personal protective equipment (e.g., barriers, machine guards) are all examples of control measures.

4. Monitoring and Review: Consistent monitoring and review of control measures contribute to the verification of their efficacy in mitigating risks within the workplace. Continuous assessment of occupational health and safety (OHS) performance, investigation and reporting of incidents, and input from employees are critical in order to identify areas requiring enhancement and to execute necessary corrective measures.

B. Occupational Health Policies and Programs

The establishment of all-encompassing occupational health policies and programs is critical for fostering a health-conscious work environment and guaranteeing adherence to regulatory obligations.

The following are essential elements of occupational health policies and programs:

1. Health and Safety Policy: Formulate a health and safety policy in writing that delineates the organization's dedication to ensuring a secure and healthy workplace, along with the obligations and responsibilities of management, staff, and administrators in upholding occupational health and safety standards.

2. Health Promotion Programs: The implementation of health promotion programs that promote healthy behaviors—including but not limited to smoking cessation, physical activity, nutrition, and stress management—can reduce the risk of chronic diseases and injuries and enhance employee well-being.

3. Implementation of Workplace Wellness Initiatives: The provision of wellness programs in the workplace, including employee assistance programs (EAPs), mental health support services, and access to preventive health assessments, can effectively mitigate psychosocial risks and

foster the psychological and emotional welfare of staff members.

4. Staff Empowerment and Safety Education: By offering extensive training and educational initiatives encompassing occupational health and safety (OHS) subjects including hazard identification, secure work methodologies, emergency response protocols, and the appropriate utilization of personal protective equipment, organizations enable their personnel to safeguard both themselves and their peers against potential dangers in the workplace.

5. Provision of Occupational Health Services: Enabling employees to utilize occupational health services, including but not limited to pre-employment screenings, medical surveillance programs, injury treatment, and rehabilitation services, promotes timely return to work outcomes and facilitates early detection and management of work-related health issues.

C. Workplace Ergonomics

By ensuring that work environments, tasks, and equipment are tailored to the cognitive and physical abilities of employees, workplace ergonomics reduces the likelihood of musculoskeletal disorders (MSDs), fatigue, and other injuries associated with ergonomics. Fundamental tenets of ergonomics in the workplace include:

1. Workspace Design: The incorporation of adjustable desks, chairs, and computer workstations into the design of workspaces to accommodate the requirements and preferences of employees contributes to the enhancement of comfort, productivity, and general welfare.

2. Task design entails the reduction of repetitive motions, ungainly postures, and excessive force in order to enhance work efficiency and quality while mitigating the risk of motor system disorders (MSDs). By implementing job rotation, task variation, and pauses, fatigue can be avoided and physical strain can be mitigated.

3. Equipment Design: The implementation of ergonomic equipment and tools, which are user-friendly, sized appropriately, and pleasant for employees, serves to mitigate the likelihood of injuries and enhance work output. Illustrative instances encompass

ergonomic controllers, keyboards, tools, and lifting aids.

4. Training and Awareness: By offering training and awareness initiatives pertaining to ergonomic principles, appropriate lifting techniques, and workstation arrangement, employers can enlighten their employees regarding the significance of ergonomics and enable them to implement necessary modifications to their work environments.

5. Ethnometric Evaluations: The performance of ergonomic evaluations on workstations, tasks, and equipment facilitates the detection of ergonomic risks and the implementation of corrective actions to enhance ergonomics and mitigate the occurrence of work-related injuries.

Ensuring organizational success, safeguarding employee well-being, and establishing a secure and healthful work environment all require efficient occupational health and safety management. Through the establishment of comprehensive risk assessment and management strategies, the development of occupational health programs and policies, and the promotion of workplace ergonomics, organizations have the ability to mitigate workplace hazards, avert work-related illnesses and injuries, and cultivate an environment that prioritizes the health, safety, and well-being of every employee.

VII.

OCCUPATIONAL HEALTH PROMOTION AND WELLNESS

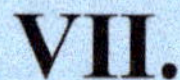

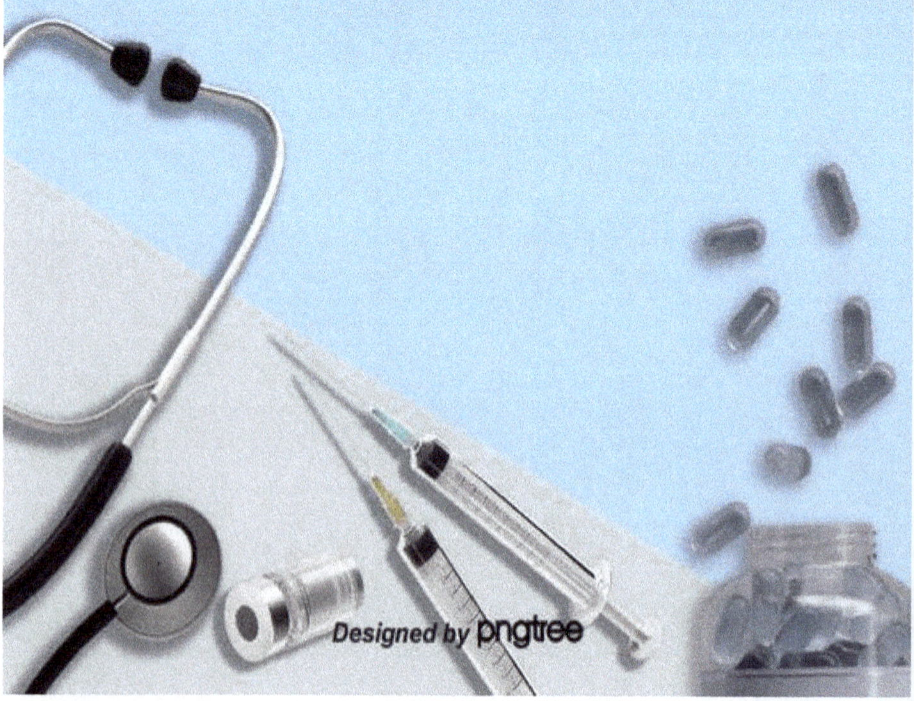

Occupational health promotion and wellness are integral components in fostering a conducive work environment, advancing the welfare of employees, and bolstering the productivity of the organization. An organization can cultivate a health and wellness culture that benefits both its employees and itself by supporting mental health and well-being initiatives, instituting health promotion activities, and providing assistance programs for employees.

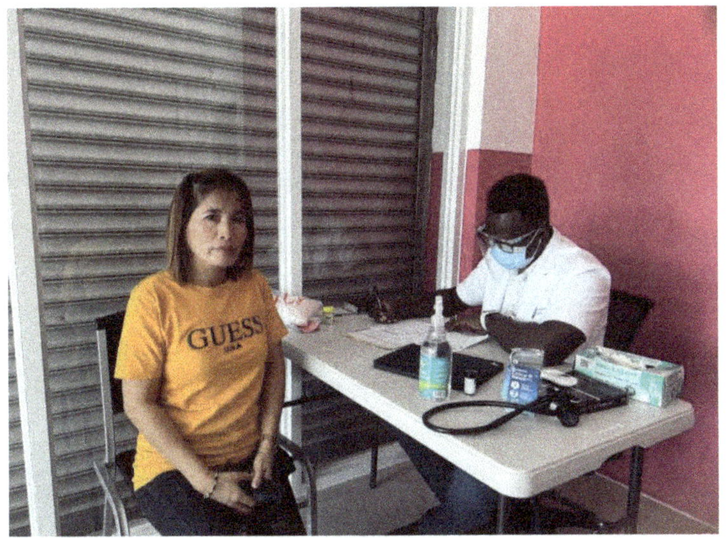

A. Health Promotion Activities in the Workplace

Health promotion activities within the workplace comprise an extensive array of endeavors that are specifically designed to enhance the physical, mental, and emotional welfare of employees. Possible such activities comprise:

1. Health Education Workshops: Implementing workshops and seminars encompassing subjects including nutrition, exercise, stress management, smoking cessation, and stress management serves to enlighten personnel regarding the merits of adopting a healthy lifestyle and furnishes them with actionable approaches to enhance their well-being.

2. Physical Activity Programs: Inspire employees to participate in consistent physical activity by organizing sports leagues, walking groups, fitness classes, and yoga sessions. Such programs have been shown to mitigate the risk of chronic diseases, elevate mood, and promote overall well-being.

3. Nutrition Programs: By offering access to nutritious food options, counseling on healthy eating, culinary demonstrations, and resources for healthy eating, these programs encourage employees to adopt nutritious eating practices, aid in weight management, and prevent chronic diseases.

4. Health evaluations: By providing onsite health evaluations, which encompass measurements such as body mass index (BMI), blood pressure, cholesterol, and blood sugar, employees are able to evaluate their overall health and detect possible risk factors that may contribute to the development of chronic diseases.

5. Wellness Challenges: The implementation of wellness challenges, including step challenges, weight loss competitions, and mindfulness challenges, serves to cultivate a sense of camaraderie among staff members and inspires them to embrace more health-conscious behaviors.

6. Health Promotion Campaigns: Initiating health promotion campaigns centered around critical health concerns, including mental health awareness, workplace safety, heart health, and cancer prevention, serves to enhance public consciousness regarding these matters and motivates personnel to modify their conduct.

7. Workplace Health Policies: The establishment of work environments that foster employee well-being is accomplished

through the implementation of health policies that encourage healthy behaviors, including but not limited to smoke-free policies, healthy vending options, and flexible work schedules.

B. Mental Health and Well-being at Work

Well-being and mental health are fundamental elements of wellness and occupational health promotion. Creating a supportive environment, minimizing stigma, and providing resources and support for employees facing mental health challenges are all components of workplace mental health promotion. Crucial initiatives comprise:

1. The implementation of mental health awareness training and education initiatives encompassing stress management, resilience development, suicide prevention, and stress management contributes to the reduction of stigma and enhanced understanding of mental health concerns within the professional environment.

2. Provision of Psychological Support Services: Employees are granted confidential assistance and access to resources to address

mental health concerns through the provision of counseling services, employee assistance programs (EAPs), and mental health resources.

3. Work-Life Balance: By implementing flexible work arrangements, telecommuting options, and paid time off, employers can foster a work-life balance that reduces the likelihood of stress-related illnesses and exhaustion and encourages employees to prioritize their mental and emotional health.

4. Stress Management Programs: The provision of stress management seminars, mindfulness training, relaxation techniques, and stress-reduction resources aids in the development of coping mechanisms and resilience among employees, enabling them to effectively navigate stressors associated with their work.

5. Implementation of Peer Support Programs: The establishment of peer support programs, mentorship opportunities, and support networks fosters a sense of community and belonging among employees by connecting them with counterparts who may be undergoing comparable difficulties.

6. Support and Communication from Leadership: Establishing a work environment that promotes open and supportive communication among leaders regarding mental health, encourages the proactive pursuit of assistance, and exemplifies self-care practices fosters a sense of worth, assistance, and empowerment among employees, thereby motivating them to give precedence to their mental well-being.

C. Employee Assistance Programs

Organization-sponsored assistance programs (EAPs) are intended to provide support to staff members who are confronted with personal or professional difficulties that have the potential to affect their health and job functioning. EAPs commonly provide a variety of services, such as:

1. Counseling Services: Offering employees and their family members confidential counseling services to address a range of work-related and personal concerns, such as mourning and loss, substance abuse, stress, anxiety, and depression.

2. Crisis Intervention: Provision of crisis intervention services and prompt assistance for personnel undergoing personal or professional emergencies, traumatic occurrences, or critical incidents.

3. Provision of Legal and Financial Assistance: Granting employees access to consultation services for legal and financial matters to aid them in navigating estate planning, debt management, legal issues, and other personal concerns.

4. Workplace Mediation: Provide mediation services and facilitate conflict resolution in the workplace to assist personnel in resolving interpersonal disputes, enhancing communication, and preserving positive professional relationships.

5. Health and Wellness Resources: Assisting employees' holistic well-being by providing resources and information pertaining to health and wellness subjects including exercise, stress management, nutrition, and work-life balance.

6. Provision of Referral Services: Facilitating connections between employees and suitable

community resources, healthcare providers, mental health professionals, and support groups in order to attend to their unique concerns and requirements.

Organizations can exhibit their dedication to fostering employee well-being, positive workplace culture, and increased job satisfaction through the implementation of comprehensive employee assistance programs.

Wellness and occupational health promotion initiatives are crucial for fostering a productive, supportive, and healthy workplace. An organization can cultivate a health and wellness culture that benefits both its employees and itself by supporting mental health and well-being initiatives, instituting health promotion activities, and providing assistance programs for employees. Investing in the health and well-being of employees yields several positive outcomes, including increased productivity, reduced healthcare expenditures, enhanced job satisfaction, and increased organizational success.

VIII.

OCCUPATIONAL MEDICINE IN SPECIFIC INDUSTRIES

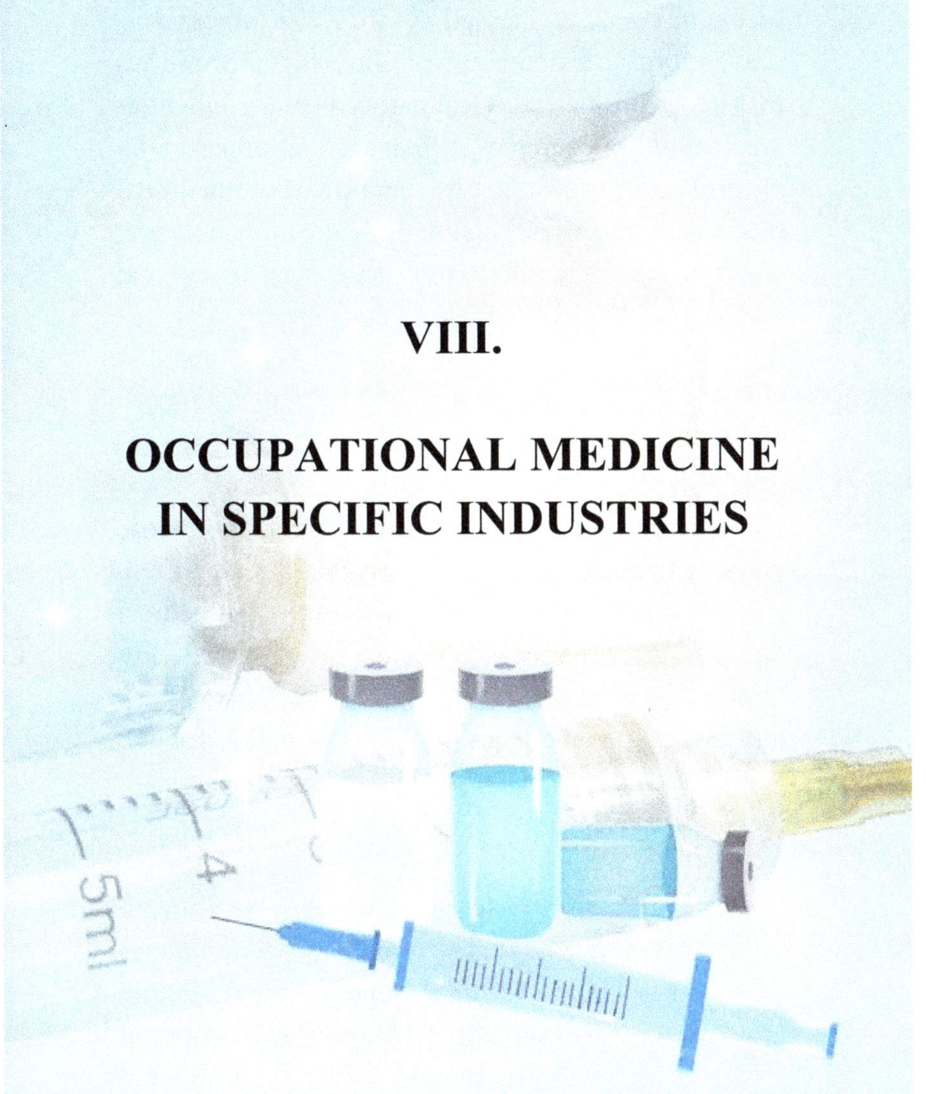

A specialized discipline of medicine, occupational medicine is concerned with the diagnosis, prevention, and treatment of illnesses and injuries that occur on the job. Occupatory health challenges are distinct for each industry on account of particular hazards and exposures. The function of occupational medicine in four distinct sectors—healthcare, construction, manufacturing, and agriculture and farming—will be examined in this paper.

A. Healthcare Industry

Healthcare is an industry that is marked by a wide array of risks, including psychological strain, occupational violence, and exposure to infectious diseases. Occupational medicine is of paramount importance in the healthcare sector as it guarantees the well-being and security of healthcare personnel. Key elements of occupational medicine in healthcare include the following:

1. Infectious Disease Control: Healthcare professionals are more susceptible to encounters with pathogens, viruses, and bacteria, among others. Occupational medicine professionals fulfill a vital function by executing infection control protocols, administering vaccinations, and delivering

personal protective equipment (PPE) training in order to mitigate the likelihood of healthcare-associated infections (HAIs) and ensure the well-being of both personnel and patients.

2. Occupational Safety: The dynamic and physically taxing nature of healthcare environments can give rise to ergonomic risks, including ungainly postures, repetitive motions, and lifting and transferring patients. By conducting ergonomic evaluations, providing instruction on secure patient handling methods, and furnishing assistive devices and equipment to mitigate musculoskeletal injuries, occupational medicine effectively tackles these risks.

3. Psychological Well-being: Prolonged work hours, substantial workloads, and exposure to traumatic incidents can substantially contribute to the stress, exhaustion, and emotional strain that healthcare professionals may encounter. Occupational medicine practitioners provide mental health support, counseling, and stress management programs to aid healthcare personnel in managing work-related stressors and preserving their health.

4. Preventive Healthcare: Occupational medicine advocates for the adoption of preventive health care practices, such as wellness programs, immunizations, and routine health screenings, among healthcare professionals. Occupational medicine contributes to the mitigation of work-related injuries and ailments among healthcare professionals by offering advice on risk factors and advocating for healthy behaviors.

B. Construction Industry

In addition to exposure to hazardous materials and accidents, electrocution, and struck-by incidents are among the most dangerous hazards in the construction industry. Occupational medicine in the construction industry is concerned with assuring the health and safety of construction workers and mitigating these risks. Key elements of occupational medicine in the construction industry include the following:

1. Safety Education and Training: Construction workers are furnished with safety education and training by occupational medicine practitioners, encompassing subjects such as

electrical safety, scaffolding safety, accident prevention, and the appropriate utilization of personal protective equipment (PPE). Construction site accidents and injuries are mitigated with the assistance of occupational medicine through the promotion of safe work practices and the dissemination of information.

2. Health Surveillance: A multitude of occupational health hazards, such as noise, pollution, asbestos, and silica, may be encountered by construction workers. Occupational medicine implements health surveillance initiatives to monitor the well-being of employees and identify potential occupational ailments, such as noise-induced hearing loss, asbestos-related diseases, and silicosis, through the utilization of medical examinations, pulmonary function tests, and hearing tests.

3. Emergency Response Planning: In order to address potential workplace incidents and medical emergencies that may occur on construction sites, occupational medicine professionals formulate emergency response plans and procedures. Occupational medicine works to mitigate the consequences of

accidents and injuries while concurrently enhancing emergency response times through the implementation of first aid, CPR, and evacuation protocols for personnel.

4. Prevention of Substance Abuse: The utilization of substances, encompassing both alcohol and drugs, which affect discernment, coordination, and decision-making, can elevate the likelihood of accidents and injuries in construction environments. To detect and resolve substance misuse concerns among construction workers, occupational medicine implements prevention programs such as counseling services, employee assistance programs (EAPs), and drug testing.

C. Manufacturing Industry

The manufacturing sector comprises an extensive array of procedures and undertakings, which give rise to a variety of occupational health risks, including but not limited to pollution, ergonomic concerns, chemical exposures, and machinery malfunctions. Safeguarding the health and safety of manufacturing personnel is the primary objective of occupational medicine in the manufacturing sector.

Key elements of occupational medicine in the manufacturing sector include the following:

1. Chemical Safety: Personnel employed in the manufacturing sector might encounter a multitude of chemical perils, encompassing vapors, solvents, metals, and acids. Occupational medicine performs exposure assessments, enforces control measures including personal protective equipment (PPE) and ventilation systems, and administers medical surveillance programs to oversee the well-being of employees and identify potential health complications associated with chemical exposure at an early stage.

2. Machine Guarding and Safety: In the manufacturing sector, incidents of machinery-related harm are prevalent, including compression injuries, amputations, and lacerations. Occupational medicine practitioners perform machine guarding evaluations, impart knowledge regarding machine safety protocols, and execute engineering safeguards with the objective of mitigating the likelihood of accidents and injuries associated with machinery.

3. Noise Management: Prolonged exposure to excessive noise levels within the manufacturing setting may result in the development of auditory disorders such as tinnitus and hearing loss. To safeguard the hearing health of employees, occupational medicine performs noise assessments, implements noise control measures including hearing protection devices and sound insulation, and provides hearing conservation programs.

4. Musculoskeletal disorders (MSDs) such as carpal tunnel syndrome, tendonitis, and low back pain among manufacturing workers may be exacerbated by ergonomic considerations, which encompass repetitive tasks, awkward postures, and manual handling of large loads. Ergonomic risks are mitigated by occupational medicine via evaluations of workstations, adjustments to ergonomic designs, and instruction on correct lifting techniques and ergonomic work procedures.

D. Agriculture and Farming

Due to environmental factors, machinery hazards, ergonomic risks, and exposure to agricultural substances, agriculture and farming are inherently hazardous industries. The primary objective of agricultural occupational medicine is to safeguard the well-being and security of agricultural laborers. Key elements of occupational medicine in agriculture include the following:

1. The safety of pesticides: Agricultural laborers face potential health hazards due to potential exposure to pesticides and other chemical substances utilized in agriculture. Medical surveillance programs, PPE evaluations, and engineering controls are a few of the control measures and control strategies that occupational medicine employs to monitor the health of workers and identify early warning indications of pesticide-related health issues.

2. Safety of Machinery: Injuries resulting from machinery operations pose a substantial menace in the agricultural sector, encompassing hazards including entanglement, crush injuries, and equipment accidents. Occupational medicine

practitioners perform machinery safety evaluations, instruct personnel on the proper operation and maintenance of equipment, and implement engineering safeguards in an effort to reduce the likelihood of accidents and injuries associated with machinery.

3. Prevention of Heat Stress: Agricultural laborers frequently encounter elevated temperatures and humidity, which elevates the susceptibility to heat-related ailments, including heat exhaustion and heat stroke. To shield employees from the detrimental consequences of heat exposure, occupational medicine employs heat stress prevention strategies such as hydration programs, shade provision, and rest intervals.

4. Prevention of Zoonotic Diseases: Agricultural laborers might encounter zoonotic diseases, including leptospirosis, brucellosis, and Q fever, which are transmitted from animals to humans. Educational initiatives and training programs are administered by occupational medicine in order to prevent zoonotic diseases. Control measures, including personal hygiene practices and vaccinations, are implemented, and medical surveillance programs are

provided to monitor the health of employees and identify potential health complications associated with zoonotic disease exposure.

IX.

LEGAL AND ETHICAL ASPECTS OF OCCUPATIONAL MEDICINE

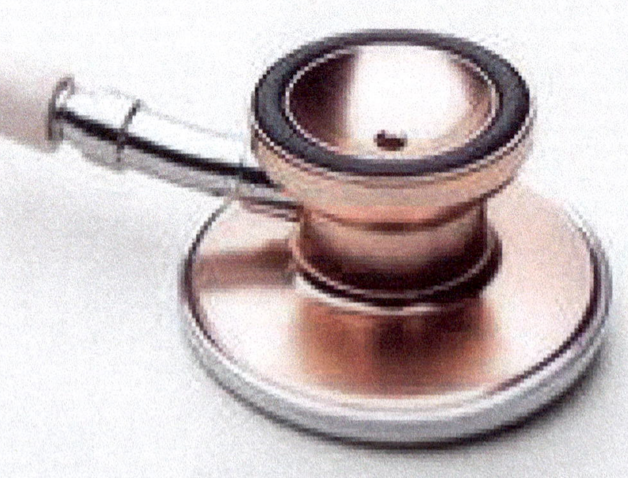

Occupational medicine is a discipline that is bound not only by legal obligations but also by ethical principles, which serve to safeguard the health and safety of workers while maintaining professional integrity and moral standards. This essay shall examine the ethical considerations and legal framework that influence the practice of occupational medicine.

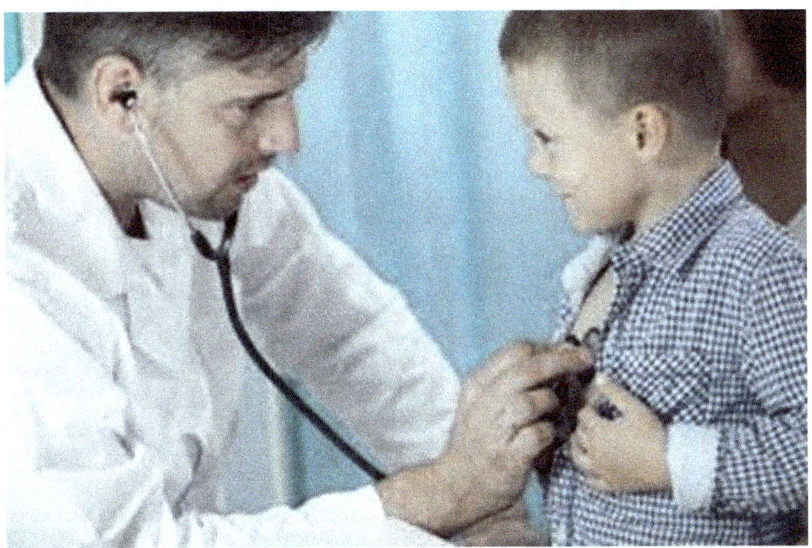

A. Occupational Health Legislation

Occupational health legislation comprises laws, regulations, and standards intended to secure the health and safety of workers and protect them from workplace hazards. While legal provisions may differ across countries, they typically comprise the subsequent fundamental elements:

1. Workplace Safety Regulations: Employers are obligated to furnish their personnel with a secure and healthful work environment in accordance with occupational health and safety legislation. Frequently, these regulations encompass training, record-keeping, hazard identification, risk assessment, and the implementation of control measures.

2. Health Surveillance Obligations: Certain occupational health laws impose a duty on employers to implement health surveillance initiatives for employees who have been exposed to particular hazards in the workplace. Pre-employment medical examinations, periodic health evaluations, and monitoring of exposure-related health effects are all potential components of these programs.

3. Worker Compensation Laws: Employees who sustain work-related injuries or ailments are entitled to financial and medical benefits under worker compensation laws. Generally, these regulations delineate the procedures

involved in lodging claims, ascertaining eligibility for benefits, and adjudicating conflicts between employers and employees.

4. Anti-Discrimination Legislation: Employers are prohibited by anti-discrimination laws from engaging in employee discrimination on the basis of genetic information, age, gender, race, disability, or disability. These legislative measures guarantee equitable access to employment prospects and safeguard employees against workplace discrimination.

5. Privacy and Confidentiality Regulations: Provisions safeguarding the privacy and confidentiality of employees' health information are frequently incorporated into occupational health legislation. Employers are generally obligated to secure consent before gathering and divulging medical information, in addition to upholding secure protocols for the storage and management of sensitive health data.

B. Ethical Issues in Occupational Health Practice

Occupational health professionals are tasked with managing a multitude of ethical considerations in their line of work, in addition to adhering to legal obligations. Such utmost professionalism guarantees the protection and welfare of employees. Several significant ethical concerns arise in the field of occupational health practice.

1. Conflicts of Interest: In order to uphold their professional judgment, occupational health professionals are obligated to preserve objectivity and independence in their evaluations and suggestions, while actively avoiding any potential conflicts of interest. This consists of abstaining from participation in activities that may exert an influence on their judgments, such as accepting gifts or incentives from insurers or employers.

2. Acquiring Informed Consent: Acquiring informed consent is a critical component of occupational health practice, particularly in situations involving health surveillance, diagnostic testing, or medical examinations. Employees have the right to be informed about the potential benefits, risks, and objectives of these interventions so that they

can make an educated choice regarding their involvement.

3. Ensuring the privacy and confidentiality of employees' health information is of the utmost importance in the field of occupational health. Occupational health personnel are obligated to maintain rigorous confidentiality protocols, divulging medical information solely to authorized parties for valid reasons, including treatment, evaluation, or compliance with legal obligations.

4. Non-Discrimination and Equity: It is the responsibility of occupational health professionals to ensure that all workers receive fair and non-discriminatory care, irrespective of their origin, social standing, or personal attributes. It is incumbent upon them to champion equitable treatment and ensure that vulnerable or marginalized groups, such as migrant workers, temporary employees, and individuals with disabilities, have access to occupational health services.

5. Professional Competence and Integrity: It is anticipated that practitioners of occupational health uphold elevated standards of

professional competence and integrity in their professional conduct. This entails maintaining awareness of the most recent optimal methodologies, complying with guidelines grounded in empirical evidence, and actively pursuing continuous education and training to augment their expertise.

6. Social Responsibility: In addition to advocating for community well-being, environmental sustainability, and social justice, occupational health professionals have a broader ethical obligation to do so. They might champion policies and procedures that place a premium on the health and safety of employees, mitigate occupational risks, and confront systemic inequities within the work environment.

Occupational medicine is an interdisciplinary field that is constrained by ethical principles and legal obligations to safeguard the health and safety of employees while maintaining professional integrity and moral standards. Occupational health professionals have the capacity to ensure the welfare of employees and foster a safer and more health-conscious work environment by abiding by occupational health legislation and incorporating ethical considerations into their professional conduct.

X.

FUTURE TRENDS IN OCCUPATIONAL MEDICINE

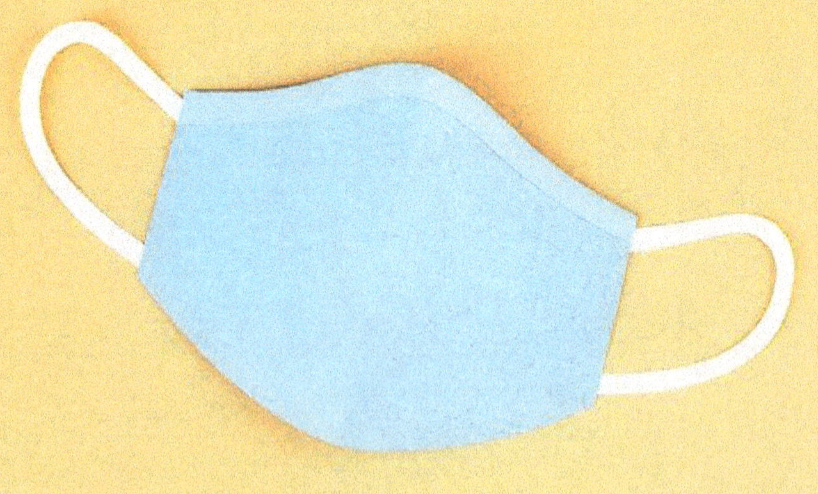

As a result of technological advancements and the complexities of globalization, occupational medicine, the medical specialty concerned with the health and safety of workers, is undergoing profound changes. The aforementioned trends are fundamentally altering the occupational health domain, introducing novel prospects and imposing distinct obstacles. This essay will examine forthcoming developments in occupational medicine, with a specific emphasis on the influence of globalization and technological progress on occupational health concerns.

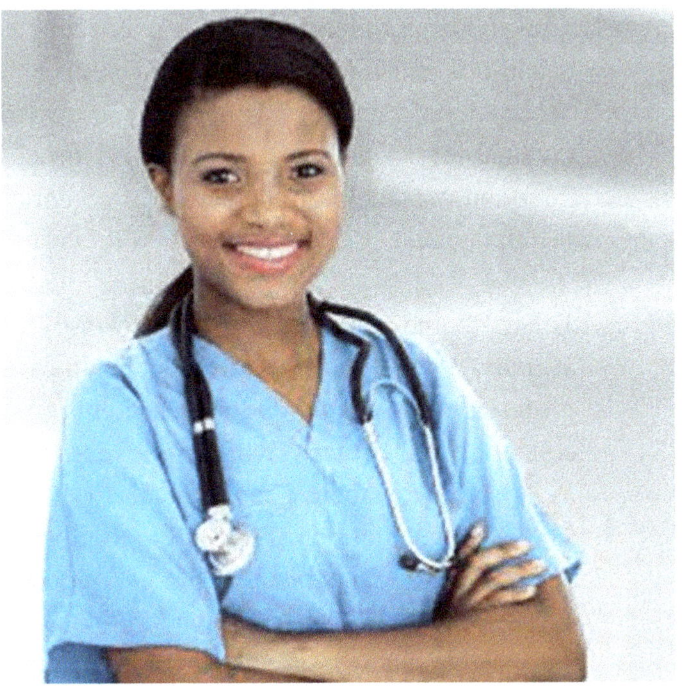

A. Technological Advancements in Occupational Health

Occupational medicine is undergoing a technological revolution that enables practitioners to monitor, assess, and manage the health and safety of employees more effectively. Among the significant developments propelling this trend are:

1. Wearable Technology: Sensor-equipped wearable devices have the capability to continuously monitor a range of health parameters, including but not limited to pulse rate, body temperature, and exposure to hazardous substances. These devices furnish occupational health professionals with invaluable data, enabling timely interventions and early detection of potential health dangers.

2. Telemedicine and Remote Monitoring: By utilizing telemedicine platforms, healthcare professionals can conduct assessments and consultations virtually with employees, i.e., irrespective of their geographical location. The implementation of remote monitoring technologies enables the ongoing surveillance of environmental conditions and the health status of employees, thereby

facilitating the timely identification of occupational hazards and encouraging proactive measures.

3. The utilization of data analytics tools and artificial intelligence (AI) algorithms enables the examination of extensive datasets pertaining to occupational health and safety. This analysis aims to detect potential hazards, trends, and patterns. Occupational health professionals can enhance the effectiveness of their initiatives, prioritize interventions, and optimize safety protocols in the workplace through the utilization of AI and data analytics.

4. The utilization of Virtual Reality (VR) and Augmented Reality (AR): Occupational health and safety training programs are incorporating VR and AR technologies to conduct ergonomic assessments, hazard recognition exercises, and immersive training simulations. These technologies augment educational experiences by providing workers with the opportunity to simulate and engage in interactive virtual environments, thereby facilitating the practice of safety protocols and risk reduction strategies.

5. Internet of Things (IoT) and Smart Sensors:
    Internet of Things (IoT) and smart sensor
    devices can automate workplace safety
    protocols, detect potential hazards, and
    monitor environmental conditions. By
    enabling real-time monitoring and control of
    workplace hazards, these technologies reduce
    the risk of occupational maladies and injuries
    and improve safety measures.

B. Globalization and Occupational Health Challenges

Enhanced cross-border mobility and interconnectedness are hallmarks of globalization, which poses distinctive hazards to occupational health and safety. Several significant challenges have emerged as a result of globalization, which are as follows:

1. The complexity of supply chains: The
    involvement of numerous stakeholders
    spanning various nations and regions in
    global supply chains presents a formidable
    obstacle in the pursuit of maintaining
    uniform health and safety standards
    throughout the entire network. Occupational
    health professionals are required to
    collaborate with international partners and

advocate for standardized health and safety practices in order to resolve the complexity of supply chains.

2. Migration and Personnel Occupational health management is confronted with difficulties through the mobility of employees, which includes migrant workers, expatriates, and temporary workers. Language and cultural barriers, as well as restricted healthcare service availability, could potentially impede the ability of these workers to protect themselves from occupational hazards and health risks.

3. Emerging Occupational Health Risks: In globalized workplaces, exposure to emerging infectious diseases, environmental contaminants, and psychosocial stressors are examples of the new occupational health risks that have emerged as a result of globalization. In order to address global health challenges, occupational health professionals must adapt to these emerging risks through the implementation of proactive measures and collaboration with international partners.

4. Regulatory Variability: Multinational corporations and global workforce management may encounter difficulties due to the variability of occupational health regulations and standards across regions and countries. Occupational health professionals are tasked with the responsibility of managing regulatory variability through diligent awareness of local regulations, active promotion of harmonized standards, and adherence to relevant laws and regulations.

5. Health Disparities and Social Determinants: Health inequities and disparities among various populations, such as laborers in low-income and middle-income nations, marginalized communities, and informal sectors, are further intensified by globalization. In order to promote equitable health outcomes for workers worldwide, occupational health interventions must effectively target social determinants of health, including but not limited to poverty, inequality, and healthcare utilisation.

The trajectory of occupational medicine in the coming years is determined by technological progress and the complexities of globalization. Occupational health professionals can enhance their ability to safeguard the well-being and safety of workers on a global scale by embracing novel technologies and adjusting to the intricacies of a work environment that is increasingly interconnected. Nonetheless, in order to confront the distinctive obstacles presented by globalization, it is imperative to foster cooperation, advocate, and maintain a steadfast dedication to advancing fair health results for every employee, irrational as to their socioeconomic standing or geographic placement.

XI.

CONCLUSION

Occupational health and safety (OHS) are critical components in safeguarding the physical and mental health of employees while maintaining a secure and wholesome workplace. Over the course of history, the discipline of occupational medicine has undergone significant development, propelled by legislative milestones, progress in health assessment, strategies for management, and an expanding comprehension of occupational hazards and diseases.

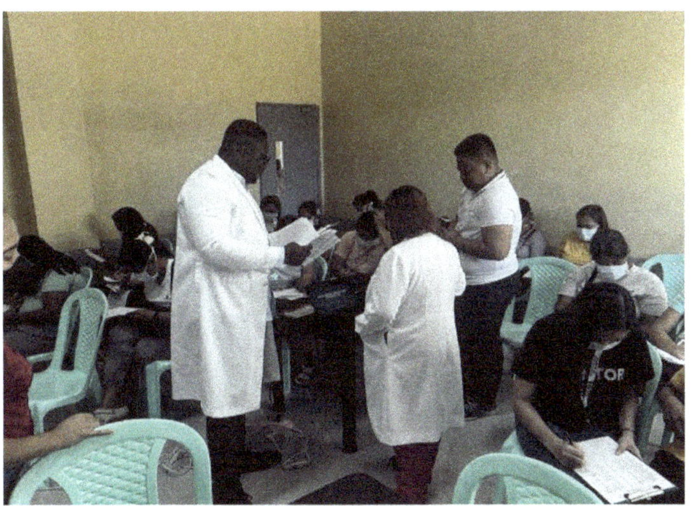

The chronicles of occupational medicine document a trajectory characterized by momentous scuffling blocks in legislative efforts to advance workplace safety and protect the rights of employees. These legislative developments have contributed to the reduction of occupational diseases and hazards and established the groundwork for contemporary OHS practices.

Occupational hazards, which encompass physical, chemical, biological, and psychosocial risks, present perils to the well-being and security of employees in a wide range of sectors. It is critical to identify and mitigate these hazards by implementing health promotion initiatives, risk assessments, and control measures. Doing so will effectively prevent occupational maladies and injuries.

Extended exposure to occupational hazards gives rise to a range of physiological and psychological disorders, including occupational maladies and musculoskeletal injuries. Intervention, surveillance, and early detection are crucial for controlling these diseases and mitigating their negative effects on employee health and productivity.

Occupational health assessments are indispensable instruments for identifying hazards in the workplace and evaluating the health condition of employees. They encompass medical examinations, physical evaluations, and health screenings. The data obtained from these evaluations is crucial for the development of targeted interventions and the implementation of preventative measures aimed at reducing occupational hazards.

A comprehensive approach to occupational health and safety (OHS) management is necessary, which includes risk assessment, hazard control, emergency preparedness, and employee training. The establishment of resilient occupational health and safety (OHS) management systems guarantees adherence to regulatory requirements, cultivates a safety-oriented organizational culture, and nurtures a more salubrious workplace milieu for all personnel.

OHS management places significant emphasis on the promotion of employee health and wellness, implementing programs that target mental well-being, health promotion, and assistance to employees. In addition to improving employee morale and productivity, wellness program investments decrease absenteeism and healthcare expenditures.

Occupational medicine expands its scope to encompass distinct sectors, where it confronts distinct health hazards and concerns. Various sectors, including manufacturing, construction, healthcare, and agriculture, rely heavily on industry-specific regulations and customized interventions to safeguard the health and safety of their employees.

Occupational medicine is influenced by ethical and legal obligations, which underscore the criticality of maintaining confidentiality, obtaining informed consent, and preventing discrimination in the management of occupational health and safety.

Recommendations for Improving Occupational Health and Safety:

1. It is imperative that governmental and regulatory entities maintain a steadfast commitment to the advancement and implementation of comprehensive occupational health and safety legislation. This will guarantee adherence to regulations and promote accountability throughout all sectors.

2. Improve Hazard Identification and Control: It is imperative for employers to consistently perform risk assessments and enforce control measures in order to alleviate occupational hazards and avert ailments and injuries in the workplace.

3. Encourage Health Surveillance: The implementation of regular health screenings and surveillance initiatives allows for the timely identification of occupational illnesses, which in turn streamlines the process of intervention and treatment.

4. Allocating Resources towards Training and Education: Fostering a safety-oriented culture and enhancing the knowledge, abilities, and proficiencies of employees, managers, and occupational health practitioners through the implementation of comprehensive training and education initiatives.

5. Promote Collaboration and Sharing of Knowledge: Fostering collaboration among various stakeholders—employers, employees, governments, and healthcare professionals—encourages the exchange of knowledge, the sharing of best practices, and collective endeavors aimed at enhancing occupational health and safety outcomes.

6. Adopt Technological Innovations: By capitalizing on technological advancements, including wearable devices, telemedicine, and data analytics, occupational health and safety (OHS) practices are consistently enhanced through improved workplace health monitoring, risk assessment, and safety training.

To achieve progress in occupational health and safety, a comprehensive strategy is necessary, which includes legislative measures, hazard detection, health monitoring, training, cooperation, and technological advancements. By placing employee well-being as a top priority and executing all-encompassing occupational health and safety (OHS) strategies, businesses can establish healthier and more secure workplaces that enhance the health, safety, and productivity of employees on a global scale.

XII.

APPENDICES

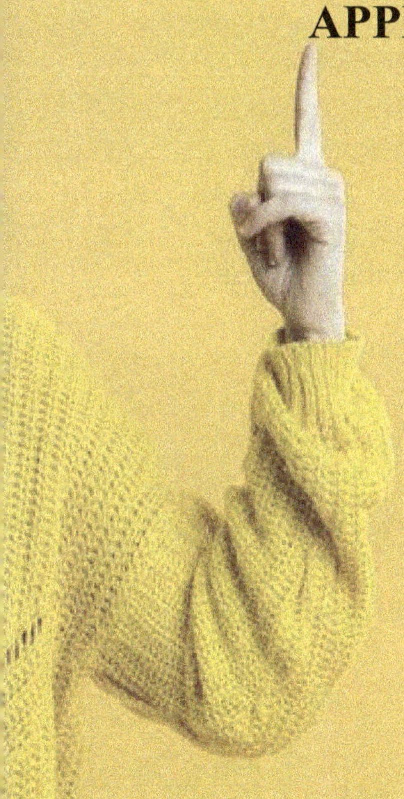

Safety Science

The Importance of Occupational Health and Safety Culture" by Mearns, et al. (2013)

Bulletin of the History of Medicine

The Origins of Occupational Medicine: History and Evolution" by Rosenstock, et al. (2006)

American Journal of Public Health

Evolution of Occupational Health Legislation in the United States" by Stebbins, et al. (2017)

Journal of Occupational and Environmental Medicine

Occupational Hazards in the Healthcare Industry: An Overview" by Smith, et al. (2020)

Occupational Medicine

Occupational Diseases: Current Trends and Future Challenges" by Jones, et al. (2018)

Journal of Occupational Rehabilitation

"Assessment of Occupational Health Risks: Methods and Applications" by Brown, et al. (2019)

Safety Science

"Effective Occupational Health and Safety Management Systems: A Review of Best Practices" by Chen, et al. (2015)

 Journal of Occupational and Environmental Medicine

Workplace Wellness Programs: Effectiveness and Implementation Strategies" by Davis, et al. (2019)

Journal of Occupational Medicine and Toxicology

Occupational Health Challenges in the Construction Industry: A Review" by Patel, et al. (2018)

Journal of Law, Medicine & Ethics

Ethical Issues in Occupational Medicine: A Comprehensive Review" by Green, et al. (2017)

Occupational Medicine

"Future Trends in Occupational Health: A Delphi Study" by Smith, et al. (2021)

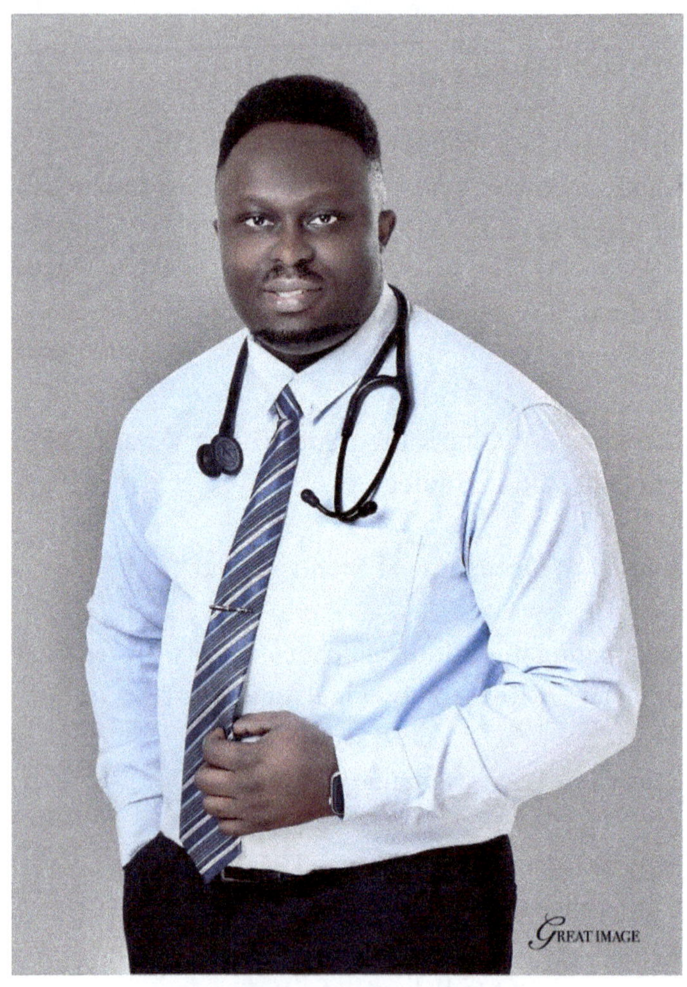

UTIPMFON SUKMAMA JIMMY, MD, MPH, MHA, DrPH, PhD
Public Health Specialist

Dr. Utipmfon Sukmama Jimmy is a highly learned and accomplished Licensed Physician, Researcher, and Writer with a distinguished career in Public Health. He finished his Bachelor of Science in Biology at Lyceum-Northwestern University in Dagupan City, Philippines. He then furthered his studies by taking up Master's in Public Health (MPH) at Virgen Milgarosa University Foundation in San Carlos City, Philippines. After completing the said degree, he proceeded with his dream of becoming a medical doctor, thereby taking up Doctor of Medicine degree in the same University in San Carlos City, Philippines. Upon completion of hismedical degree, he successfully passed the Physician Licensure Examination of the Philippines and obtained his PRC License to practice as a registered Physician.

As a Medical Doctor, he has been with a number of hospitals in the Philippines such as the Wesleyan University-Philippines Hospital, Cabanatuan city, Philippines and has worked as a Medical Transcriptionist at Dr. Gloria D. Lacson General Hospital previously. As an accomplished Medical Doctor, he never forgets to share his expertise by being an Industrial Lecturer at Wesleyan University-Philippines, Cabanatuan City, Philippines, under the College of Nursing and College of Medicine.

Furthermore, Dr. Jimmy is a Public Health Specialist; he obtained his Doctor of Public Health degree, Major in Health Promotion and Education from Angeles University Foundation in Angeles City, Philippines. More so, with a deep-rooted passion for improving patient care and ensuring optimal hospital operations, Dr. Jimmy pursued and successfully obtained a Master in Hospital Administration degree from the prestigious Wesleyan University - Philippines, Cabanatuan city, Philippines. Belonging to the school of thought that believes learning never ends, Dr. Jimmy went on to pursue the Doctor of Philosophy in Public Administration degree at Panpacific University, Urdaneta City, Philippines. With a solid foundation in medical expertise and comprehensive understanding of healthcare management principles, Dr. Jimmy has consistently demonstrated exceptional leadership skills and an unwavering commitment to delivering excellence in healthcare services. Through extensive experience in both clinical practice and administrative roles, Dr. Jimmy has developed a unique skill set that encompasses medical knowledge, strategic planning, financial management, and effective communication.

Driven by a genuine desire to positively impact the healthcare industry, Dr. Jimmy remains dedicated to improving healthcare outcomes and shaping the

future of healthcare administration by doing
extensive research.